The Miracle of Water Therapy and Oil Pulling

A Beginners Guide to Ancient Yogic Remedies

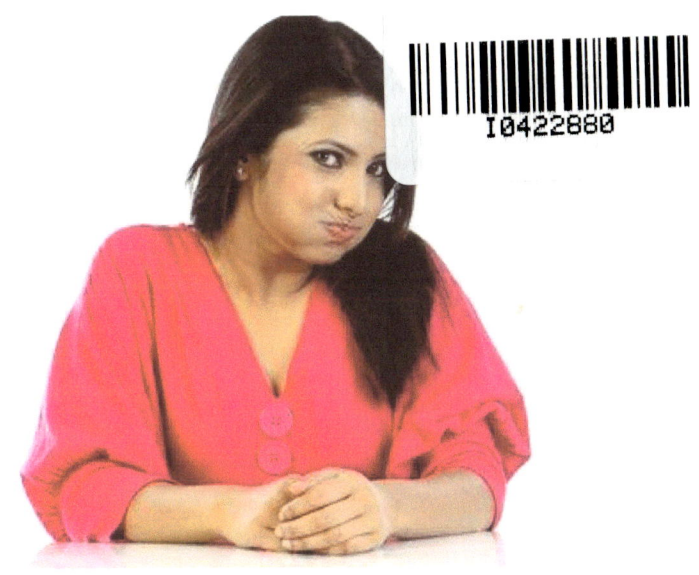

Dueep Jyot Singh

Health Learning Series

Mendon Cottage Books

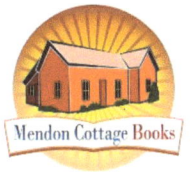

JD-Biz Publishing

Disclaimer

The information is this book is provided for informational purposes only. It is not intended to be used and medical advice or a substitute for proper medical treatment by a qualified health care provider. The information is believed to be accurate as presented based on research by the author.

The contents have not been evaluated by the U.S. Food and Drug Administration or any other Government or Health Organization and the contents in this book are not to be used to treat cure or prevent disease.

The author or publisher is not responsible for the use or safety of any diet, procedure or treatment mentioned in this book. The author or publisher is not responsible for errors or omissions that may exist.

Warning

The Book is for informational purposes only and before taking on any diet, treatment or medical procedure, it is recommended to consult with your primary health care provider.

Our books are available at

1. Amazon.com
2. Barnes and Noble
3. Itunes
4. Kobo
5. Smashwords
6. Google Play Books

Table of Contents

Introduction

Being very interested in alternative medicine forms like Ayurveda and being taught yoga as a part of our Academic curriculum, in our student days, I soon began to understand why the ancients in the East considered yoga to be an integral part of their lives. This book is going to introduce you to some of the more common ancient natural healing traditions practiced in the Indian subcontinent since ancient times.

I was talking to an American audience about alternative Indian medicine, when I spoke about Ayurveda and yoga. A friend immediately said, "But that is religious, and is based on Hindu practices."

I would like to clear up this point once and for all. These practices are definitely not based to people belonging to one religion. Besides, the people who wrote these exercises and rules for right and proper living, and practiced them millenniums ago were Aryans and they gave this knowledge in their religious and spiritual books to the people of India who were practicing Hinduism.

Practicing Hinduism? What do I mean by that?

Consider Hinduism at that time to be a way of life, practicing nonviolence and following the wise teachings of the ancient ones. It is now a full-fledged religion, incorporating those same beliefs, traditions, and way of life in their manner of living and being. The ancient knowledge of those wise ones are now being practiced, as set down in the Vedas and the Puranas.

I am definitely not a Hindu, but since childhood, I and my Hindu, Christian, Mussalman, Buddhist, Sikh and Jain Friends did all these yogic exercises every morning, during school assembly, and we never believed them to be part of a religious tradition belonging exclusively to the Hindus.

Our teachers were sensible enough not to let even an inkling of this controversial idea blossom in our infantile, suspicious and susceptible minds, because that would mean that 17% of the students would immediately have their parents yelling "keep religion out of academics. This is unacceptable. "

This is an extremely touchy subject in the East.

And because we considered these exercises to be part of PT, 15 minutes of this healthy workout kept us healthy and happy throughout our childhoods and youth. We never knew that they were yogic exercises!

According to us, we were keeping healthy, in a natural manner. We definitely did not chant Hindu hymns while doing these exercises.

That in itself would be anathema Maranatha to anybody not a Hindu, including I.

 So the idea that this universal healing tradition is limited to just one peoples, is definitely wrong, and it has been started by some lazy minded people, who would rather find excuses not to do a thing rather than work out.

So here am I –not a Hindu!- telling all my friends all over the globe how they can keep healthy, through different natural remedy practices, which have been in vogue for centuries in the Indian subcontinent.

These practices are going to include oil pulling, which is getting to be extremely popular in the West today, and also water therapy.

All this information was taken by me from an experienced Ayurvedic doctor, so that all the information that is being given to you has been time tested and has been recommended by him. But before that, you would want to know a little bit more about the terms, which I am going to be using in this book.

What is Ayurveda

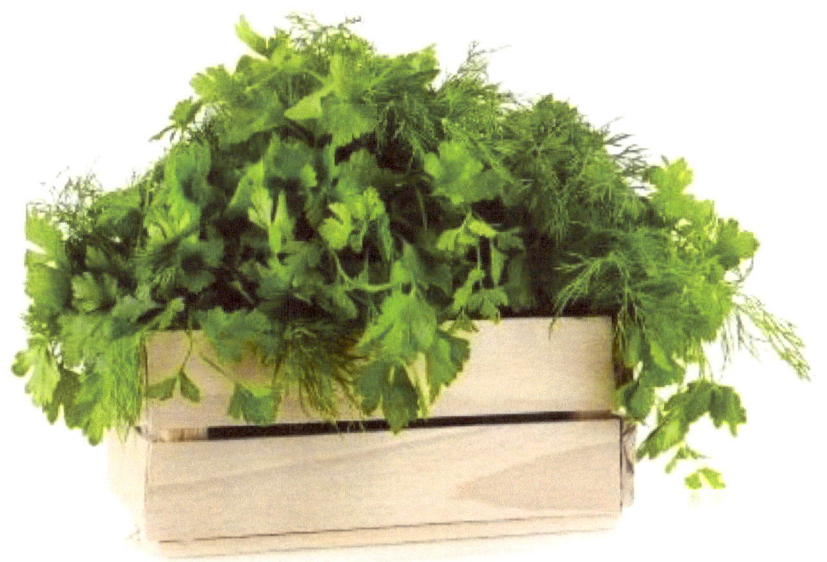

Natural products including the use of herbs and spices are a part of Ayurvedic treatments.

Ayurveda is a traditional system of alternative medicine, practiced by the ancient Hindus millenniums ago. This is based on spiritual, emotional, physical and mental harmony through meditation, natural medicine, herbal remedies, change in diet and lifestyle and yogic poses and breathing.

What Is Yoga?

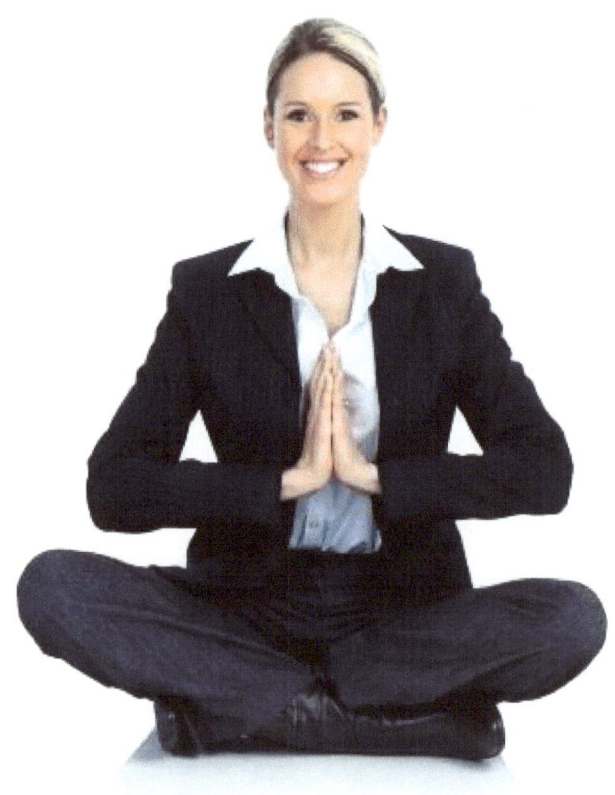

Yoga is an ascetic ancient Hindu discipline, which is spiritual, and includes meditation and breathing in different postures of the body and which is now being practiced to relax your heart, body and spirit.

Many people in the West have now discovered yoga, to be an astonishingly effective manner in which they can meditate, and de-stress themselves. This is also a natural way which you can keep healthy and tension free. More and more researchers in the West are also looking at the efficacy of Ayurveda as a form of alternative medicine, because it relies on natural remedies instead of chemicals, artificial-based drugs. Also, this medical practice takes care of your problem, through natural remedies which go to the root of the matter and help cure you.

Oil Pulling

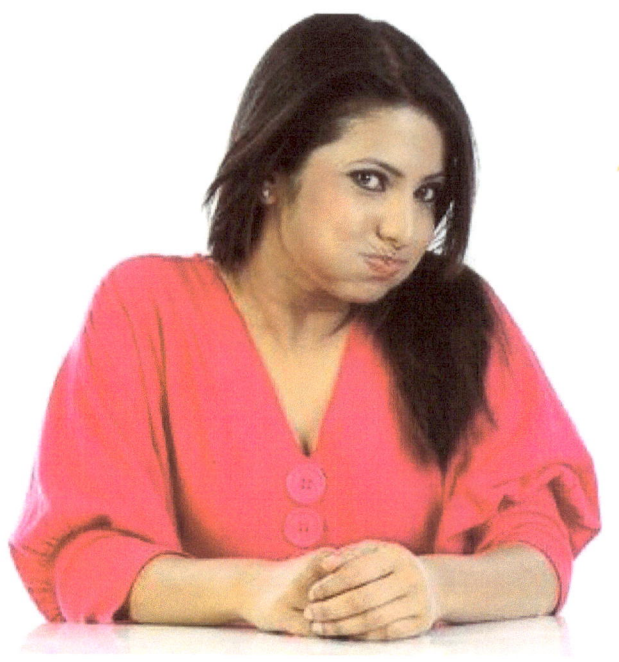

I knew all about water therapy, but when somebody suggested oil pulling to me as an effective ancient healing process, I immediately went to my Ayurvedic friend, philosopher, and guide.

He then told me that yes, this process has been in vogue for millenniums, and many people do not know about it. Consider that to be Oil Sucking, because the term "oil pulling" can also bring up a vision of the extraction of oil from seeds or from the seabed! Semantics.

So now I am going to tell you all about Oil Sucking. You are going to put some oil in your mouth, and suck it for a while. This is considered to be an effective way of which you can get rid of a number of ailments, and this is known as the Oil Sucking Remedy Procedure.

Procedure

You are normally going to use a natural oil, for this procedure. It is done in the morning. I would suggest using coconut oil, sunflower oil, peanut oil, or any other refined oil. Wash your mouth out. This is normally done before breakfast. Now take one tablespoonful of this oil, – about 10 mg – and place it in your mouth.

The taste of raw refined oil in your mouth is an acquired taste, so you may feel just this bit taken aback, the first time you taste it. Now shut your mouth, up tight, and swish the oil, all around your mouth. You are allowing the natural saliva to mingle in this oil.

For people who are still wondering how to do this, just imagine that you are substituting oil instead of your mouthwash. You swish Listerine around in your mouth, after brushing your teeth, do not you. That keeps your mouth and breath fresh. So now, instead of Listerine, we are swishing our mouths with one tablespoonful of oil. Make sure you are sucking that oil and "chewing" it, with your teeth.

Do this for 20 minutes every day.

I asked my friend to demonstrate this method to me. His way of "chewing oil" reminded me very much of a cow chewing the cud, with their exaggerated chin movements. I managed to keep back a smile. But he does this for 20 minutes every day, and he is in his 70s, young, youthful looking, and hale and hearty. So this is definitely going to work for you too.

This chewing procedure is going to encourage the production of saliva and that is what is needed. Also, this manages to draw all the toxins and poisons, in the body, through the mucous membranes of the mouth.

In about 20 minutes, that oil, which is being chewed so vigorously is going to get diluted, white in color, and is also going to get polluted and contaminated with the toxins. Spit out that oil, and then wash out your mouth thoroughly.

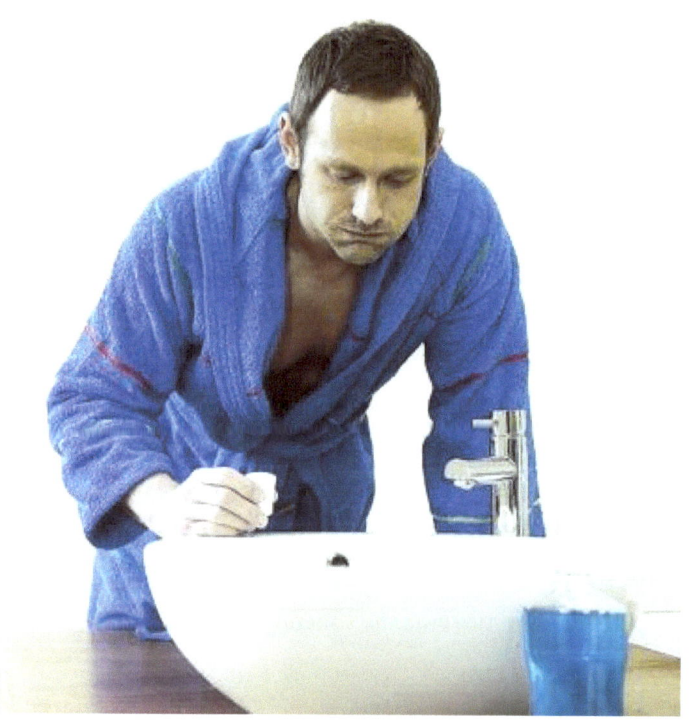

Do not swallow the oil under any circumstances because it is full of your own toxins!

Brush your teeth again and rinse out your mouth, because that oil is going to have microbes, which are not naturally present in your system. Besides, this rinsing is going to clear up your mouth. You may want to put some water up your Nasal passage and blow it out, – as if you are blowing your nose, during a cold, – during this time. This is going to help clear your sinuses and get rid of any obstructions in your nasal passage.

When to Do Oil Pulling

The best time to do the oil pulling is in the early morning, before your breakfast. It is only on an alternative medicine doctor's recommendation, that he may suggest you do this twice a day, especially if you are suffering from chronic conditions. But for "normally" healthy people like you and me and Deepak Chopra, oil pulling once a day, in the morning when you wake up is going to be amazingly effective, and is going to keep all of us healthy.

If you are going to do oil pulling, twice a day, make sure that you do it on an empty stomach. That means 2 hours before you have your dinner, when your last meal has been semi-digested.

Believe it or not, this is guaranteed effective for curing minor ailments, especially in their initial stages, in 3 to 4 days. However, chronic ailments are going to be healed over a longer period of time, which can take up to one year. But just calculate – 20 minutes per day, to help heal yourself, with one tablespoonful of oil. Is it not worth it?

Tips

Do not leave this procedure half way, just because you think that it is not helping you. It is doing its magic work, and you will soon see the visible results, in your improved state of health.

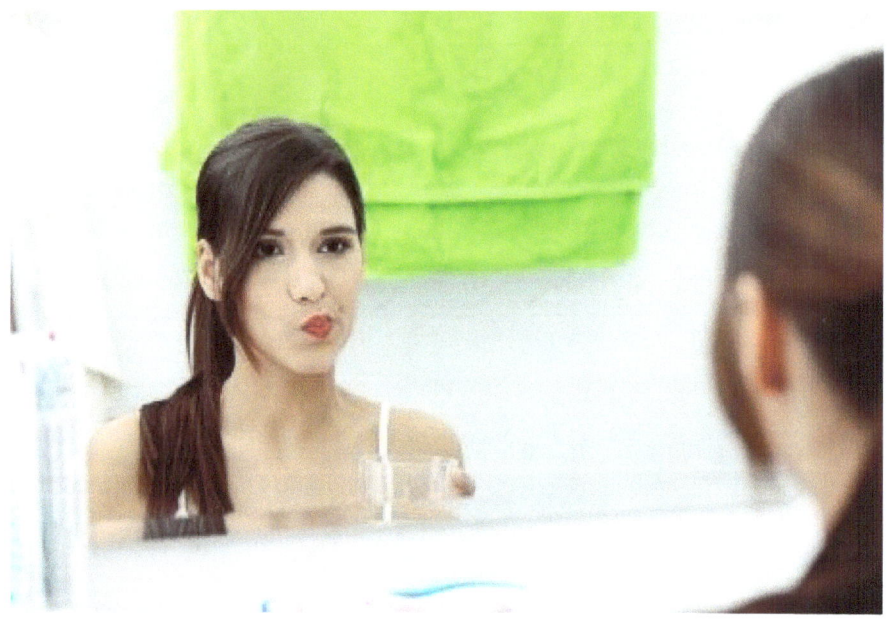

Yep, oil pulling is best done in the bathroom!

One of my friends told me that she had a feeling that her ailing state had been aggravated, ever since she started doing oil pulling. And that made her stop. Now this is a very important point. You may "feel" that some of your symptoms may grow more visible, especially if you are suffering from a number of ailments, both new and chronic. For example, you may feel an increase in temperature. Do not get terrified and leave this healing process, because your body is getting used to a new natural system to cure it from toxins and other poisons in your body.

You are soon going to see your symptoms dying away, and your ailments healing themselves. This reassurance should be enough to tell you that this process works, naturally beneficially and effectively. The aggravation of symptoms temporarily was just your body's way of telling you that it is now on its road to healing.

Ailments cured by Oil pulling

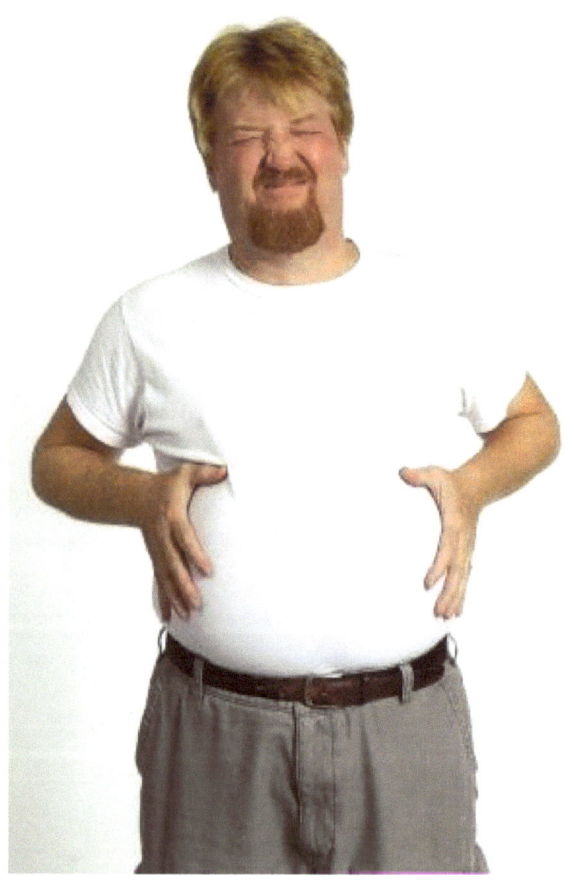

Tummy Problems Can Be Cured through Oil Pulling

Oil pulling is considered to be the panacea for a number of ailments, but here is a list of some of the ailments for which this has been proved efficacious.

Teeth ailments, including shaking teeth and gum problems, headache, problems in the blood, bronchitis, heart problems, urinary problems, liver problems, thrombosis, lung, stomach, insomnia, skin problems and osteoporosis can be helped/cured by getting rid of the toxins in your body through oil pulling.

I wonder why nobody is doing any research on oil pulling help preventing tumors from growing. In fact, I want scientific researchers to come up with scientific data, which encourages skeptics, and thus makes them open to the use of oil pulling, especially if they are suffering from tumors. So much suffering would be cured by humans, if they looked at natural healing processes. That includes alternative medicines and natural remedies.

Unfortunately, the majority of human beings are cynical by nature and skeptics by instinct. That is why they are not going to try out anything new unless somebody has shown them reams of scientific proof by scientists who have wasted huge amounts of money on proving something which has already been guaranteed effective by people half a world away, millenniums ago.

The skeptics are definitely not going to believe something which was said by the ancients ages ago, because they are often under the mental conditioning of "old remedies are quack remedies, and I cannot get cured without scientific technology, especially chemical-based drugs curing me."

These are the sort of people who I want to benefit by this book. Remember that there are many things to heaven and earth, and even if this process is not supernatural like Hamlet's ghost, it is an earthbound practice, and has been in use in ancient times by people who were not bothered much about doctors or scientific researchers!

I got rid of the dark circles under my eyes, with the help of this oil pulling. Also, I made sure that I ate plenty of greens, so that I do not suffer from possible anemia, and also stopped too many late nights. Early to bed and early to rise for two days, after a light dinner, and oil pulling for four days, and no more dark circles. So I do not look like a panda anymore.

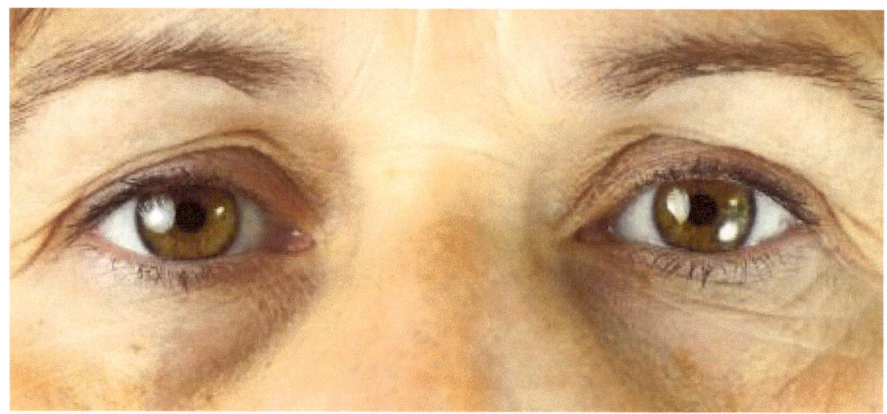

Dark circles can be due to anemia, lack of sleep, and also less essential nutrients in your diet.

Oil pulling also improved my general health, energy levels, concentration levels, appetite and enthusiasm for life. Not bad results with one tablespoonful of oil every morning.

I asked him why he did not recommend mustard oil for oil pulling. He said that many people do not going for mustard oil, because it smells so terribly. But that is his first choice, especially when you are looking for something to keep your mouth disease-free. It also prevents your lips from chapping and your throat from growing hoarse and dry. Best of all, you can eat as many sour things as you want without they having a bad effect on your teeth.

So you may want to try mustard oil, if you want a clear voice and a tough jaw! Good for men, but I do not want to be a lantern jawed female, so I stick to coconut oil.

Water Therapy

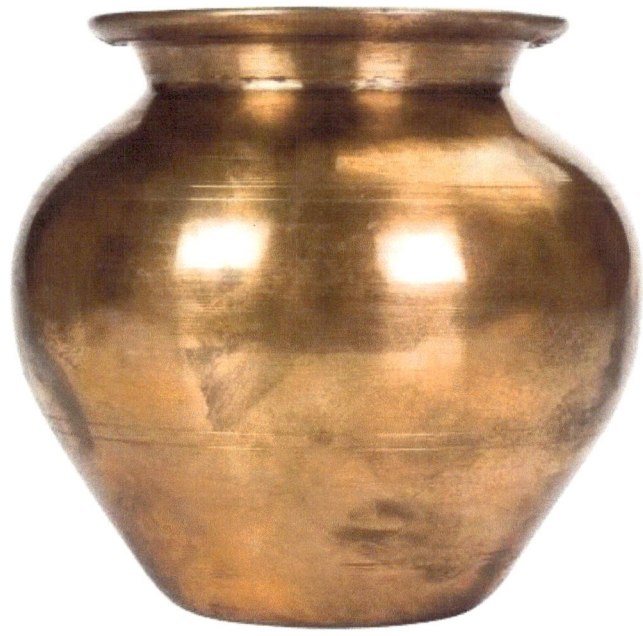

Along with oil pulling, there is another therapy, which I have found extremely effective, especially as it just uses water to help cure me.

Any pure water is going to do. But you need a copper utensil. Now, what has a copper utensil to do with water therapy? It has something to do with the mineral and the ions present in copper, and Incorporated in the water, which are going to benefit the body. As I do not quite trust the water supply in our area, I boil the water and allow it to cool. Then I put it in the copper utensil and leave it overnight.

This is the water, which is going to be used for water therapy, early in the morning, when I wake up. Do this first thing in the morning, without washing out your mouth beforehand.

Take eight handfuls – about 250 g of water – in your cupped hands and drink this down slowly. You can also sip this water directly from the copper utensil. Now get up and walk about hundred steps or so. This is to allow the water to percolate throughout your system. It is also going to activate your digestive system, and you will need to go to the bathroom. This shows that your kidneys and your liver are functioning properly.

 Hundred steps means pacing all around the inside of my home and garden for about 7 to 8 minutes. I mapped out that area by counting the steps. Do that and you know how many times, you need to go around your living room, bedroom, kitchen and garden!

40 steps is a hundred feet, so hundred steps is about 250 feet, because one step is .4 foot. 50 feet is 20 steps. This should give you an estimate on how much you need to pace every day.

This is a guaranteed effective cure for constipation. It is also considered to be a good cure for headache, piles, chest problems, eye problems and other systemic ailments.

This water therapy is considered to be one of the reasons why so many people lived long and fulfilling lives, in ancient times. The scientific explanation is that that water got rid of the toxins in the body, and the walking exercise after that make sure that you did not lead a sedentary lifestyle. Unfortunately, a large number of us, including me, cannot be made to walk, because it is such a bore. But thanks to this necessary part of water therapy, I will get the incentive to walk around a bit, and possibly get rid of some cellulite too at the same time.

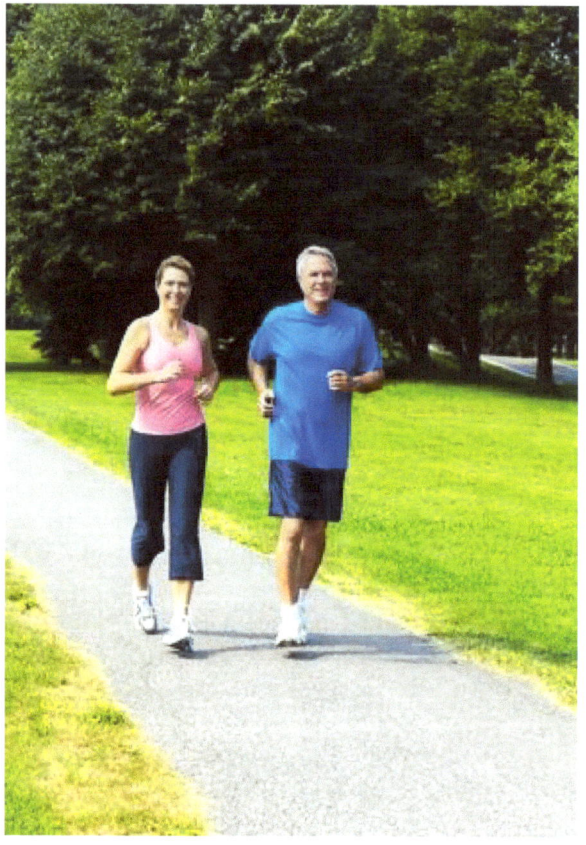

Some people may find themselves going to the bathroom a bit too often when they start this water therapy, because after all they are drinking water early in the morning. The system is not used to that. They may also find themselves suffering from mild dysentery. But this is going to disappear into three days, because your system is now used to a water intake every morning.

People suffering from joint problems or gastroenteritis problems should try out this water therapy three times in a day. They can reduce it to one after a week.

You can drink this water two hours after you have had a meal.

Water Therapy through Nostrils - Neti

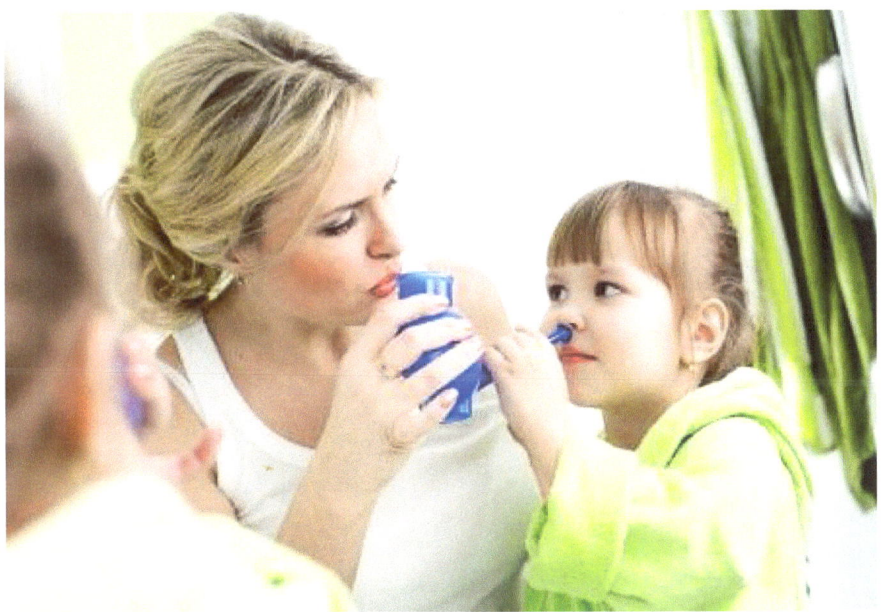

Now, now, I am going to tell a procedure where you are not going to drink the water through the mouth, but you are going to "drink" it through your nostrils. This is considered to be guaranteed effective to clear out sinus problems and other infections in your nose and mouth. It is also supposed to be extremely good for eye problems, especially to strengthen your vision. My doctor friend who still has black hair, even though he is in his 70s, attributes no graying of hair to this water therapy every day.

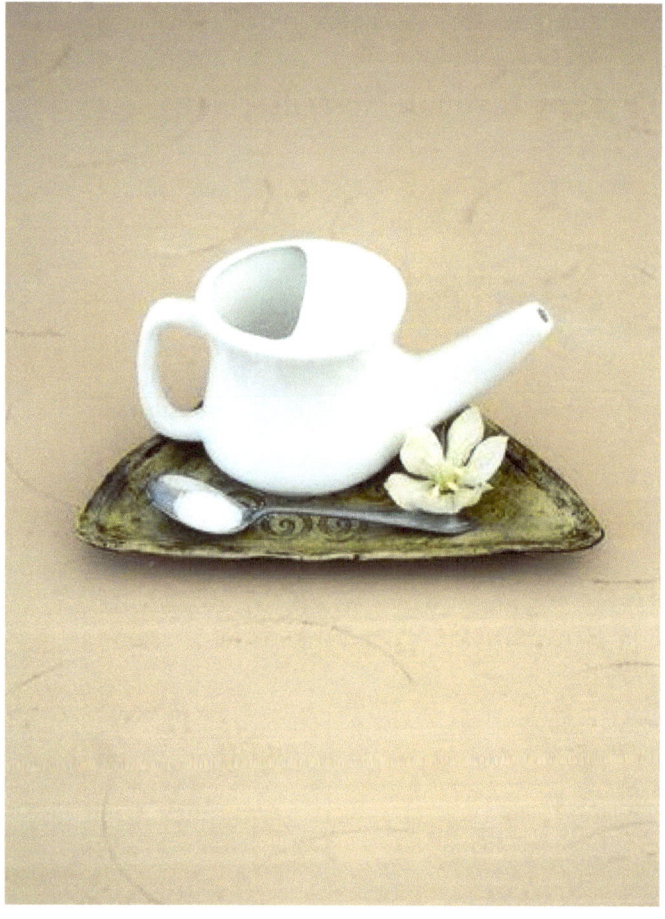

This is a fragile modern porcelain pot. The traditional Netis are normally made up of copper. They look like spouted kettles.

You may want to warm the water up a little bit, in the winter, especially as you would not want to snort in cold water, would you.

Here, you are not going to be using the copper utensil. Instead, you are going to be using a utensil with a spout called a Neti Lota – literally utensil for cleansing. You can consider this to be nasal irrigation, practiced by the ancients in yoga.

Try this out, especially if you are living in a contaminated and polluted atmosphere. This clears out your sinuses and is beneficial for all those people who are working in elements fall of dust and pollution. Mayo clinic doctors recommend this process for getting rid of chronic chest and sinus problems.

Himalayan Salt Is Best

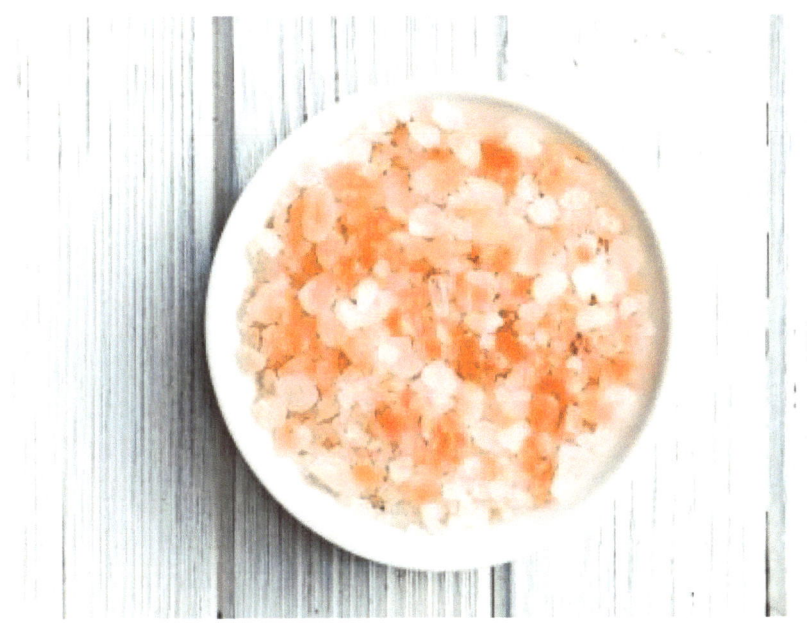

You normally put 1/8 teaspoonful of powdered Himalayan salt in water. You do not use very cold water or warm water in this exercise. This is because you are looking for a fluid which closely approximates the natural fluids already present in your body. I suggest Himalayan salts, because it is a natural salt, and is milder than sea salt. It is pinkish in color and is mined in mines in Khivra – Pakistan, and also in salt lakes in Arizona, and in Denmark.

Cooks love the salt for culinary purposes. It is healthy and has lesser amounts of iodine.

350 mL of warm water can do with 3/4 teaspoons of Himalayan salts. But you may want to change the ratio of the salts, because the sensitivity of your mucous membranes especially in your nose depends from person to person. Try with a lesser amount of salt, in the initial stages, especially when you are practicing with a Neti for the first time.

You are going to pour this liquid through one nostril, and allow the water to pour out from the other nostril. People practicing this for the first time have a problem with that water going down their throats. Been there seen that! I found it rather disgusting, because I felt that some of the waste from my nose, including the dust had gone down my throat and that thought itself was rather sickening.

So you need to close your throat passage. That is done by saying GNNNNN or krrrrrrrrr nasally – a throaty growl from the bottom of your throat – while you are irrigating your nose.

In the ancient yogic lifestyle tradition, this water cleansing was done every morning, when you took your bath, and brushed your teeth. You can practice this more often, if you are living in an atmosphere full of fall utensil, especially in the city, or you are suffering from sinus problems or even a letter allergy problems like hay fever.

I saw somebody practicing Neti in her garden, allowing the water to flow on the path. But then she was doing it in the open air. So why not.

Buying the Right Neti Pot

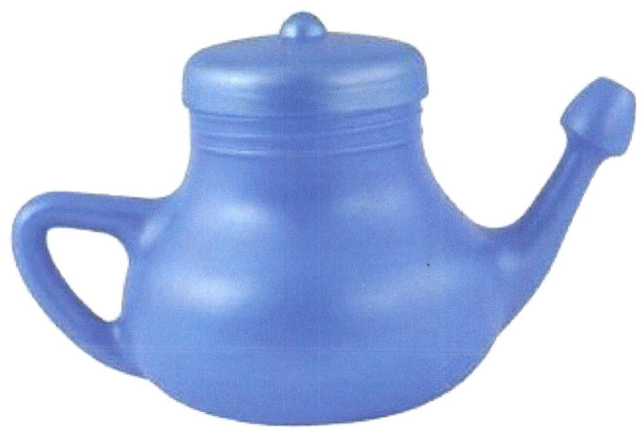

Should you go in for a porcelain one? Why not, though I am always afraid of it breaking. I have a traditional copper one, but stainless steel ones are also getting to be more and more popular in the market today.

How to Use a Neti Pot

Fill up your pot with well mixed salt and water. Open your mouth wide and take in a deep breath. This is another way of closing your throat passage. This is also going to prevent water getting into your throat or in your mouth.

I do not bend over the sink, because it is going to "worry" my neck. I normally use it under a shower, so that the water can flow on the bathroom floor, without any problems.

You may take one or two times to get used to irrigating your nestled passages with salty water, because after all, you are putting a metal spout up your nostril and allowing the water to flow out from the other nostril. But a little bit of this cleansing, and you are going to find yourself refreshed, your nasal passages clear and unclogged, and your eyes and ears feeling fresh and alive.

Now put the cone gently into your right nostril, and inhale slowly, so that water is drawn up into your nostril. Keep your left nostril closed with one finger, during this drawing up of water.

Now bend your head slowly and forward. Till it to the left so that you allow the water to flow out from the left nostril, which you release, the moment you start tilting your head.

Your chin, as well as your forehead should be at the same angle and level. You will need to experiment a bit to see which degrees of tilting works for the water to flow out. The water is going to take a little bit of time to flow out. Keep breathing all this time slowly and gently through your mouth.

Once the water is flowing out, keep your head steady at that level and remember it for tomorrow! Just keep the pot moving to keep the water flow pouring in your right nostril.

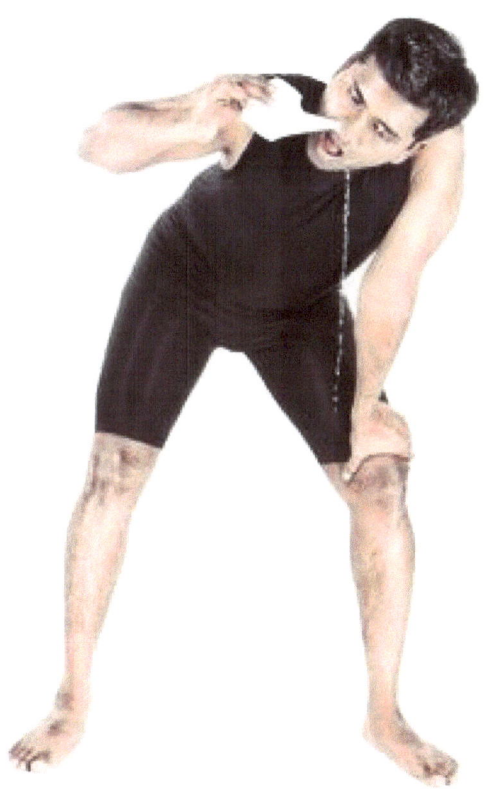

Once this has been done, remove the spout, raise your head and let all the water flow out, by blowing gently, through your nostrils.

Repeat the same procedure for your left nostril. You need to keep half the pot's amount of water in the initial stages for each side. Once you have got used to this procedure, you can use one part of water for each side.

If you find water not flowing out naturally through your nostrils, it is time to see a doctor and see if your nasal passage is not blocked.

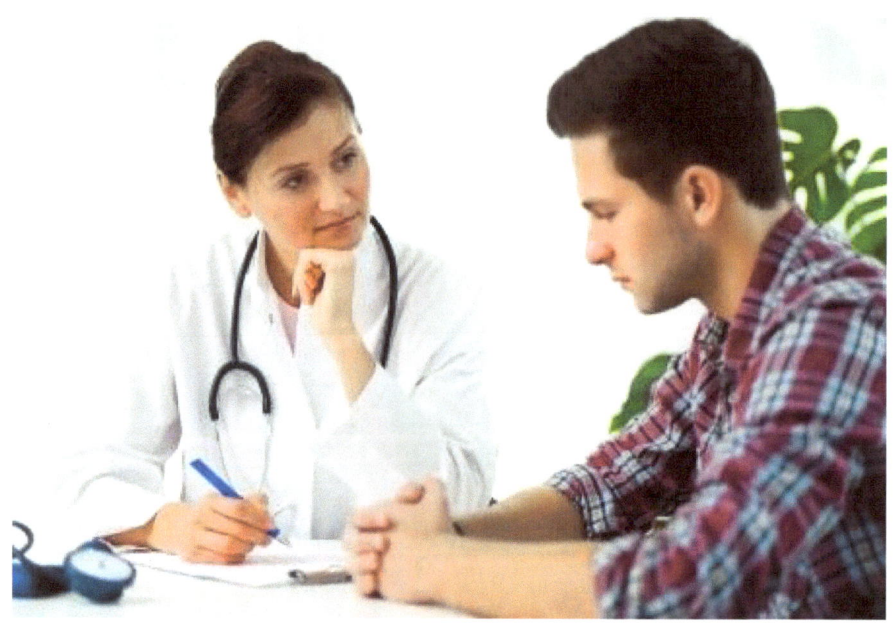

Keep your nostrils open when you are blowing out the last vestiges of water. After you have done this nasal irrigation and cleansing remember to dry out your nose thoroughly. This is also a yoga exercise called *Bhastrika Kriya*.

This is done by bending your head forward, and blowing out like the bellows of a Smith (*bhastrika*)through your nostrils in a nose blowing process so that all the water is removed. You can also tilt your head left and right while blowing out. Hold a towel under your nose when you are doing this water removal, moving your head in all directions.

Remember to rinse out your neti lota with water after use.

Benefits of Neti -based Water Therapy

This water therapy method removes all the infectious microorganisms, pollutants, and dirt from your nasal passages.

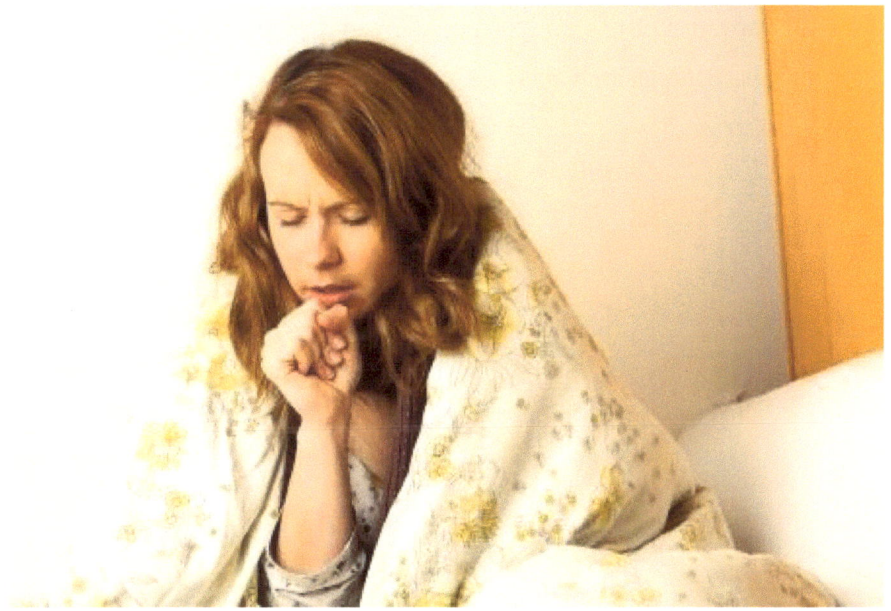

People suffering from chronic cold can find themselves with a healthy system, thanks to the salt water irrigation. It is also excellent for blocked noses.

People were suffering from bronchial problems, chronic sinusitis, and red and dry throat, eyes and noses are going to be benefited by this therapy. This is also considered to be a good way to keep your mind relaxed and tranquil.

Precautions during Water Therapy.

Some of these lifestyle tips are necessary to make sure that your water therapy is effective in curing you. Stop drinking cold drinks and foods made up of refined flour. Avoid fatty items included fried stuff. Reduce the spices in your diet. You may want to add more vegetables and fruit to your diet.

Water therapy also means that you are going to reduce your coffee, tea, alcohol, tobacco, recreational drugs and processed food intake, including ice cream and sodas.

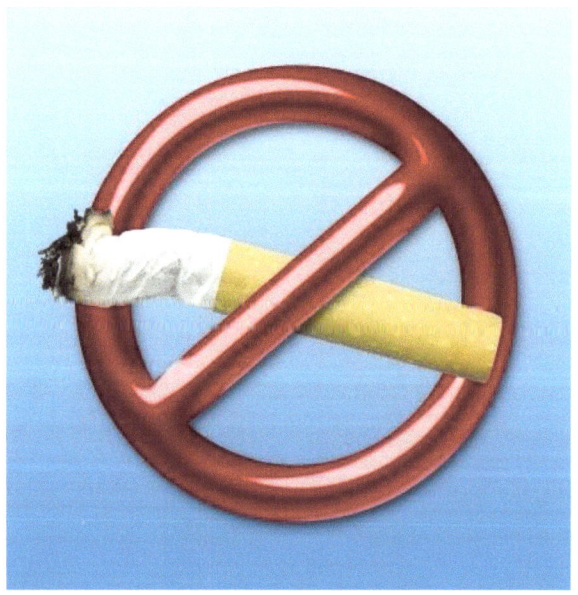

Well, this was the lifestyle, followed by the ancients who did not bother much about food with artificial preservatives and were more interested in eat healthy, eat natural.

It is said that a healthy person drinking three – four glasses of water every morning is never going to fall sick. Nevertheless, I would not advise it, because too much water at one time can lead to water retention and water logging. So just drink that much of water, which you think removes the early morning thirst, first thing in the morning.

Drink water or fresh juice as often as you feel thirsty throughout the day. Do not eat anything four hours before you go to sleep, especially fruit like apples.

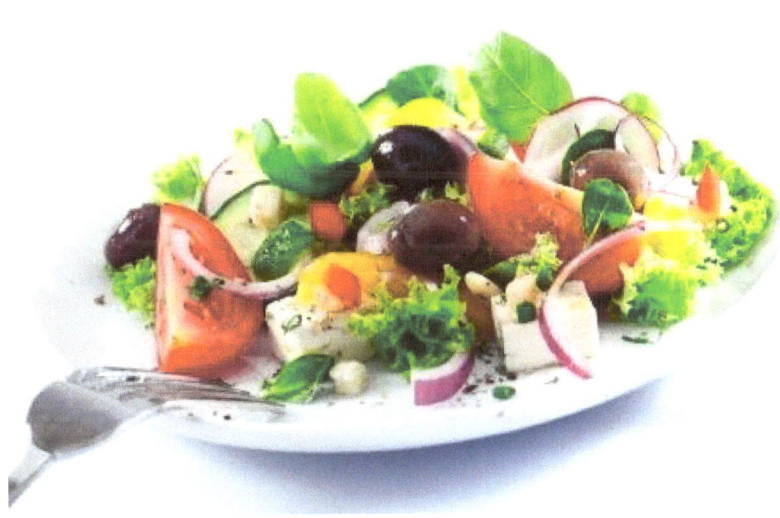

Lots of greens, and fresh organic grown food help keep you healthy.

The Japan-based Sickness Association tried this water therapy on people suffering from diabetes and blood pressure. They found positive results, in one month and relief from chronic constipation and gas in just 10 days. They are now trying this on cancer patients and TB patients. They have found healthy benefits in six months of this therapy.

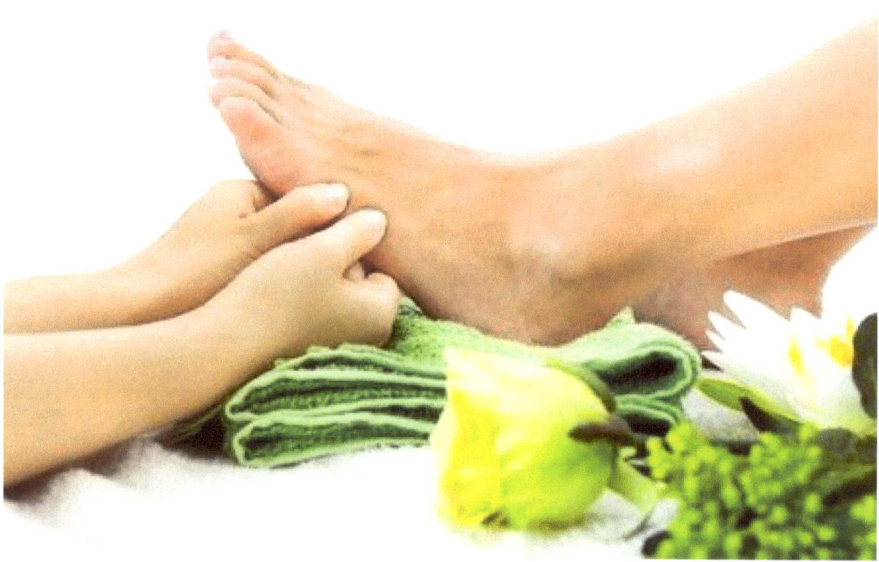

According to the Indian Health Association, this therapy is based on proven science. The toxins accumulated in the body during the last 24 hours can be done through this procedure. It also cleans out your stomach. That means that the chances of sicknesses are reduced, because you do not have any potentially infectious material allowed to decay in your stomach. I think this is a very logical explanation.

If you are using the nasal water therapy process to get rid of eye problems like myopia and hypermetropia and want to get rid of those glasses, you can try associated supporting exercises. You can consider this to be acupuncture exercises where the pressure points in your heels toes and the padded area beneath your toes are massaged with warm oil.

Do this by massaging the first and largest" Thumb" toes, and the area underneath them, before you move on to the other toes. This concentrating on the thumb toe and massaging it with oil every day improves your eyesight. The ancient Chinese knew it. And that is why they used this acupuncture pressure point to heal ailments of the eye for millenniums.

Pressure points for improving Eyesight

This was another remedy, told to me by an herbalist. Wash your face, after you have had your meals. Wash your hands **and do not wipe them**. Then rub the palms of your hands together, so that they feel a bit warm. Now place these warm hands gently over your eyelids and rub them slowly over your eyes. After that, these warm hands are rubbed all over the face.

Now I am going to be pressing pressure points with my index finger and my middle finger, while my ring finger, my thumb and my smallest finger [called Pinky in the East] are left to wave gracefully in the air.

Press your index finger and middle fingers over your eyes in the direction of nose to ear, seven times. This is going to help get rid of your glasses, even though it is going to take up to 10 months to a year. That is because this natural healing is a slow process. And the pressure points need some time to understand they are being requested to get moving.

Do not do this if your eyes are red, swollen up or are infected.

You can also try rubbing your hands together to get them warm, placing them on your cheeks and then moving your hands towards your eyes and then to your temple. He asked me to chant this autosuggestion – my eyes are getting better and better every day, in every way. They are getting healthy and more attractive too. I enjoyed this positive autosuggestion.

This rubbing off the palms and the fingers have been known since ancient times to be the collection of power and when you do that, and place it over parts of your body, it is going to benefit you.

Conclusion

I hope this book has given you plenty of information about that very interesting natural curing procedure, oil pulling, and water therapy. The Chinese, Oriental, Indian and other ancient Eastern civilizations have been using these methods for millenniums to keep them healthy, longer living and youthful looking. So enjoy the benefits of natural remedies and therapies, live long and prosper.

Author Bio

Dueep Jyot Singh is a Management and IT Professional who managed to gather Postgraduate qualifications in Management and English and Degrees in Science, French and Education while pursuing different enjoyable career options like being an hospital administrator, IT,SEO and HRD Database Manager/ trainer, movie scriptwriter, theatre artiste and public speaker, lecturer in French, Marketing and Advertising, ex-Editor of Hearts On Fire (now known as Solstice) Books Missouri USA, advice columnist and cartoonist, publisher and Aviation School trainer, ex- moderator on Medico.in, banker, student councilor ,travelogue writer ... among other things! One fine morning, she decided that she had enough of killing herself by Degrees and went back to her first love -- writing. It's more enjoyable! She already has 48 published academic and 14 fiction- in- different- genre books under her belt.

When she is not designing websites or making Graphic design illustrations for clients , she is browsing through old bookshops hunting for treasures, of which she has an enviable collection – including R.L. Stevenson, O.Henry, Dornford Yates, Maurice Walsh, C.N.Williamson, Sapper, Bartimeus and the crown of her collection- Dickens "The Old Curiosity Shop," and so on... Just call her "Renaissance Woman" collecting herbal remedies, acting like Universal Helping Hand/Agony Aunt, or escaping to her dear mountains for a bit of exploring, collecting herbs and plants, and trekking.

Check out some of the other JD-Biz Publishing books

Health Learning Series

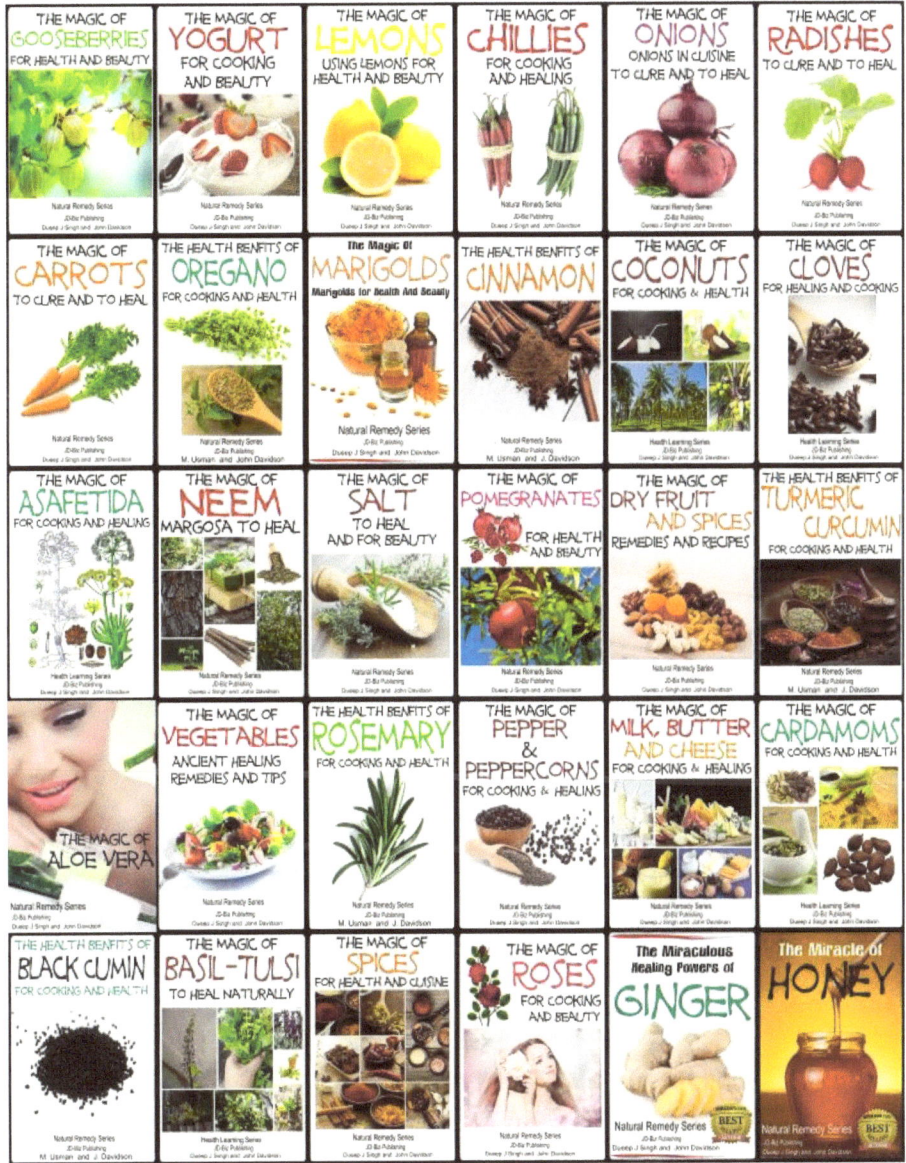

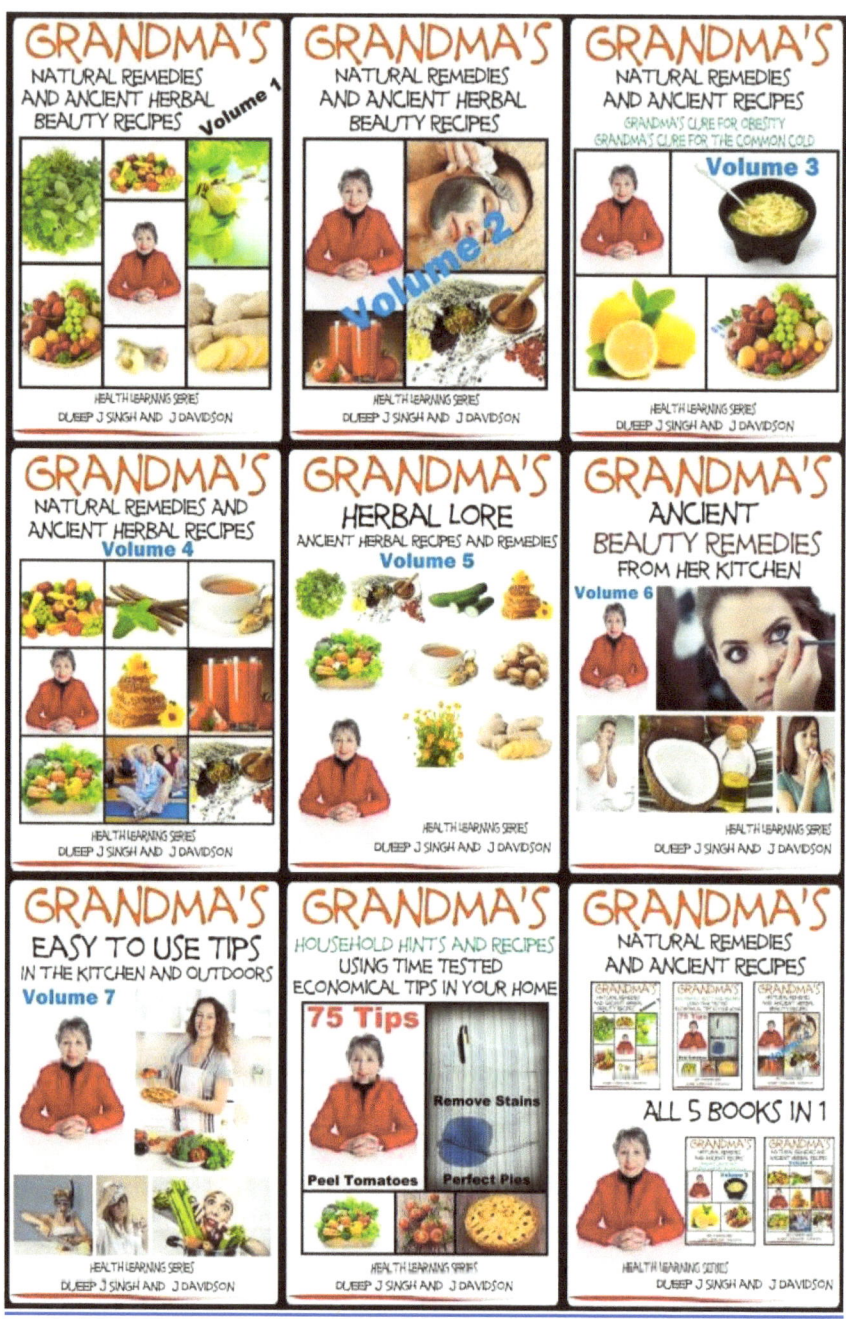

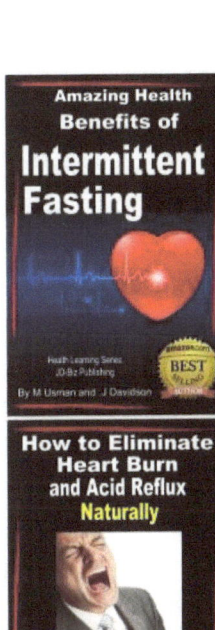

Amazing Health Benefits of Intermittent Fasting
Health Learning Series
JD-Biz Publishing
By M Usman and J Davidson
BEST SELLING

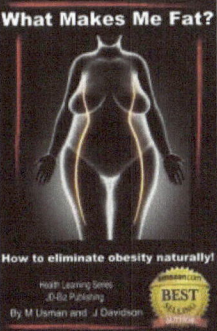

What Makes Me Fat?
How to eliminate obesity naturally!
Health Learning Series
JD-Biz Publishing
By M Usman and J Davidson
BEST SELLING

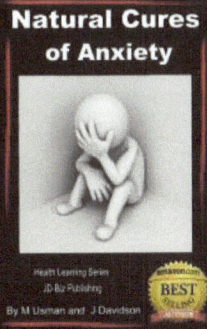

Natural Cures of Anxiety
Health Learning Series
JD-Biz Publishing
By M Usman and J Davidson
BEST SELLING

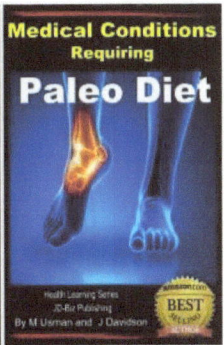

Medical Conditions Requiring Paleo Diet
Health Learning Series
JD-Biz Publishing
By M Usman and J Davidson
BEST SELLING

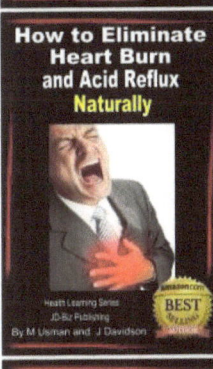

How to Eliminate Heart Burn and Acid Reflux Naturally
Health Learning Series
JD-Biz Publishing
By M Usman and J Davidson
BEST SELLING

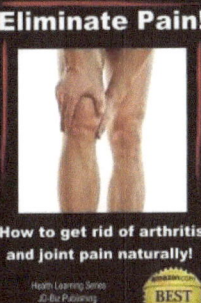

Eliminate Pain!
How to get rid of arthritis and joint pain naturally!
Health Learning Series
JD-Biz Publishing
By M Usman and J Davidson
BEST SELLING

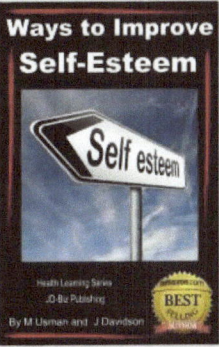

Ways to Improve Self-Esteem
Health Learning Series
JD-Biz Publishing
By M Usman and J Davidson
BEST SELLING

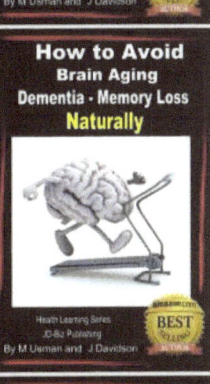

How to Avoid Brain Aging Dementia - Memory Loss Naturally
Health Learning Series
JD-Biz Publishing
By M Usman and J Davidson
BEST SELLING

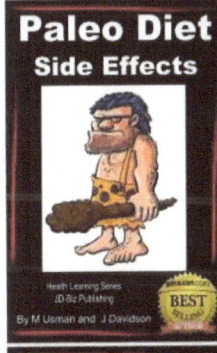

Paleo Diet Side Effects
Health Learning Series
JD-Biz Publishing
By M Usman and J Davidson
BEST SELLING

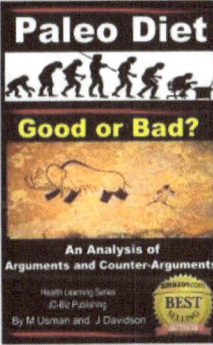

Paleo Diet Good or Bad?
An Analysis of Arguments and Counter-Arguments
Health Learning Series
JD-Biz Publishing
By M Usman and J Davidson
BEST SELLING

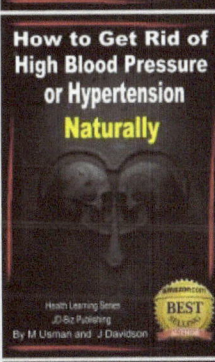

How to Get Rid of High Blood Pressure or Hypertension Naturally
Health Learning Series
JD-Biz Publishing
By M Usman and J Davidson
BEST SELLING

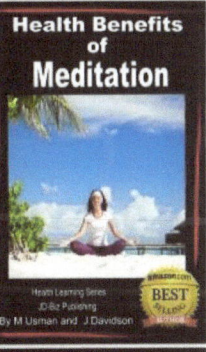

Health Benefits of Meditation
Health Learning Series
JD-Biz Publishing
By M Usman and J Davidson
BEST SELLING

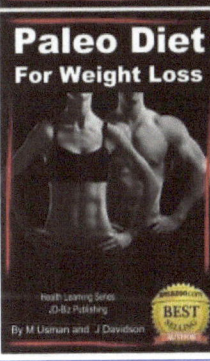

Paleo Diet For Weight Loss
Health Learning Series
JD-Biz Publishing
By M Usman and J Davidson
BEST SELLING

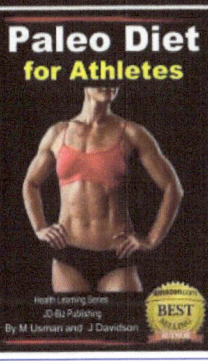

Paleo Diet for Athletes
Health Learning Series
JD-Biz Publishing
By M Usman and J Davidson
BEST SELLING

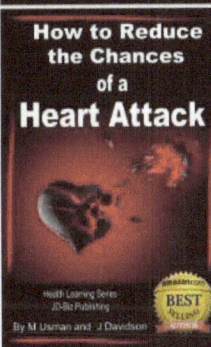

How to Reduce the Chances of a Heart Attack
Health Learning Series
JD-Biz Publishing
By M Usman and J Davidson
BEST SELLING

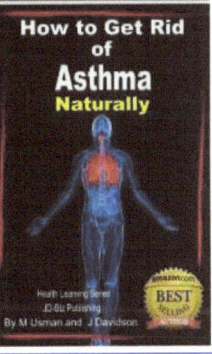

How to Get Rid of Asthma Naturally
Health Learning Series
JD-Biz Publishing
By M Usman and J Davidson
BEST SELLING

Amazing Animal Book Series

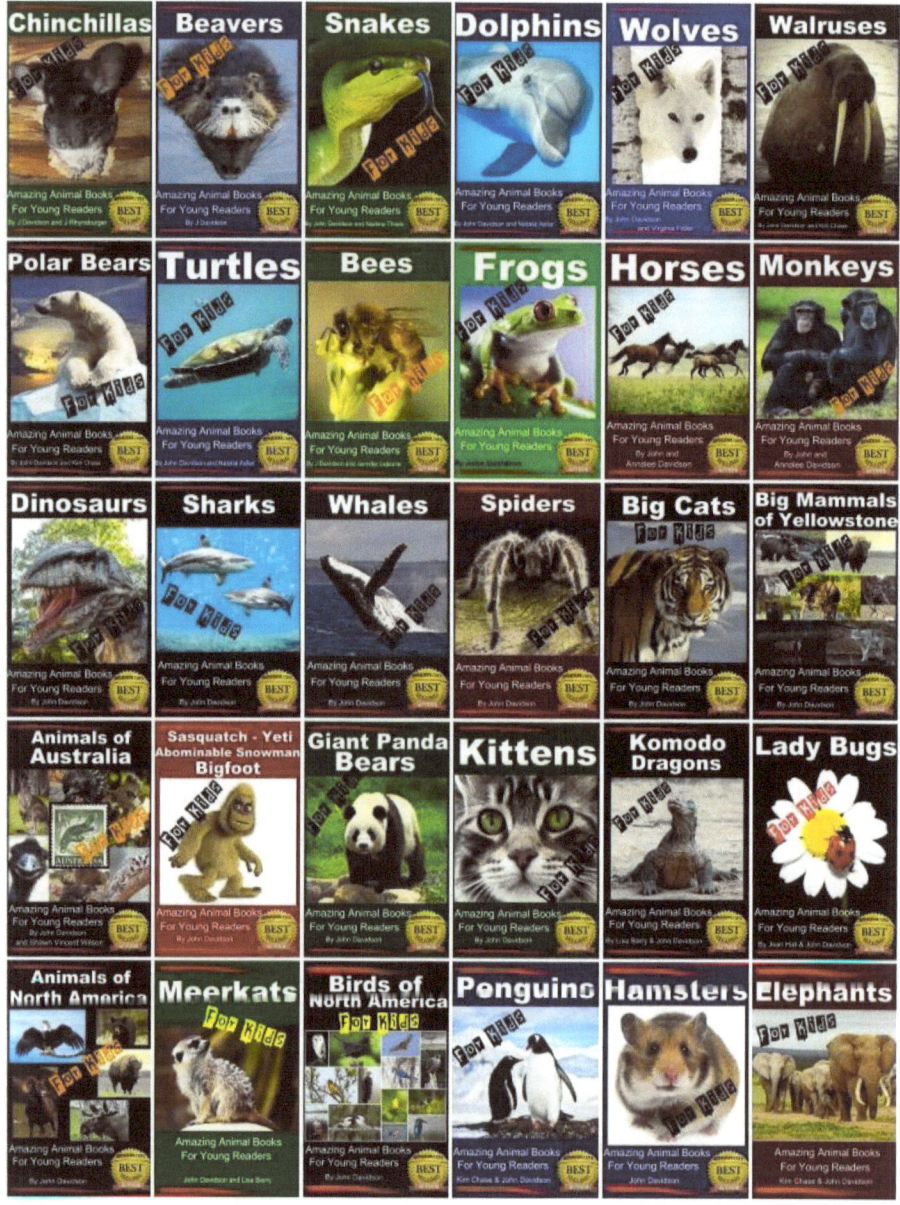

Learn To Draw Series

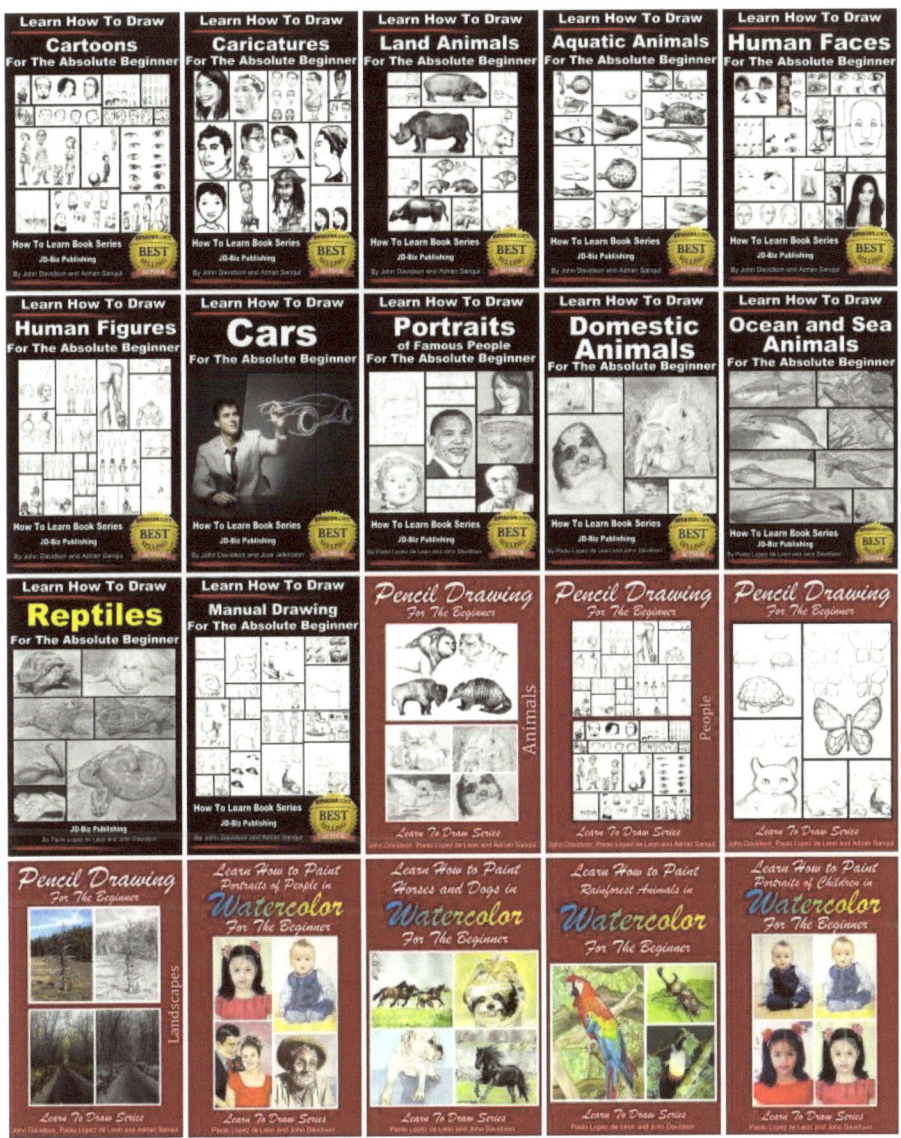

How to Build and Plan Books

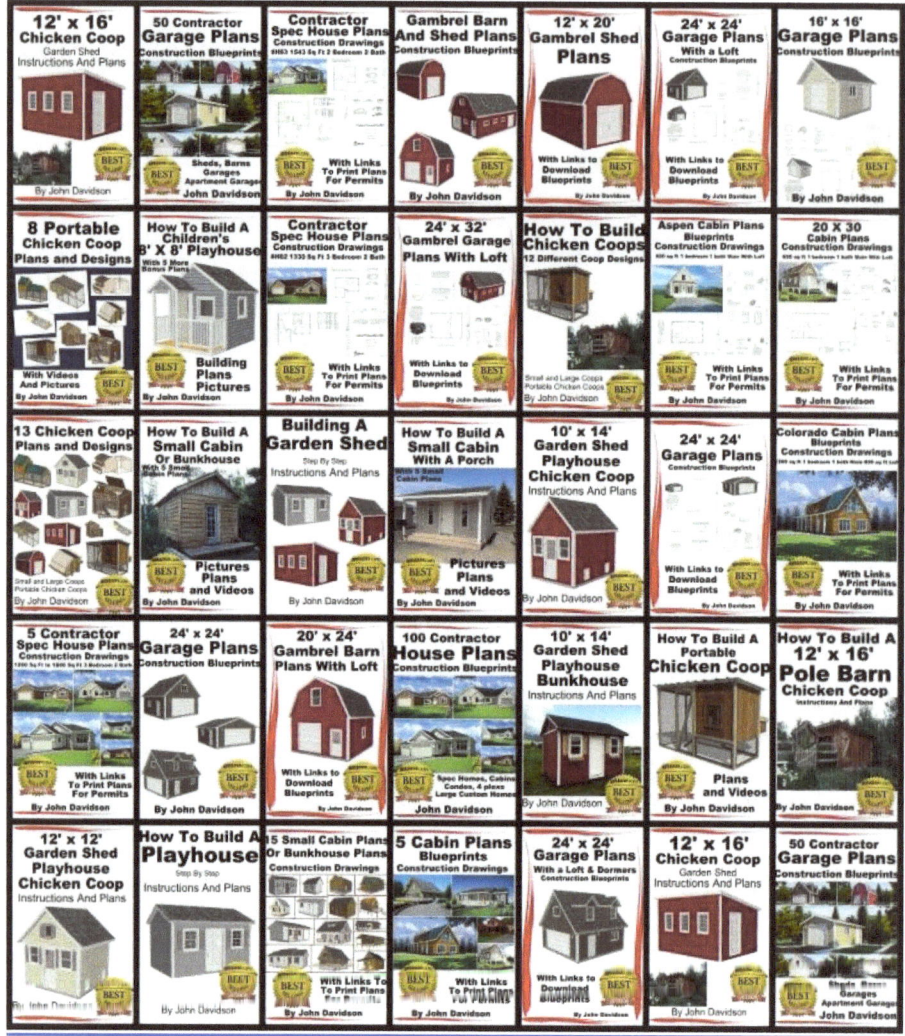

Entrepreneur Book Series

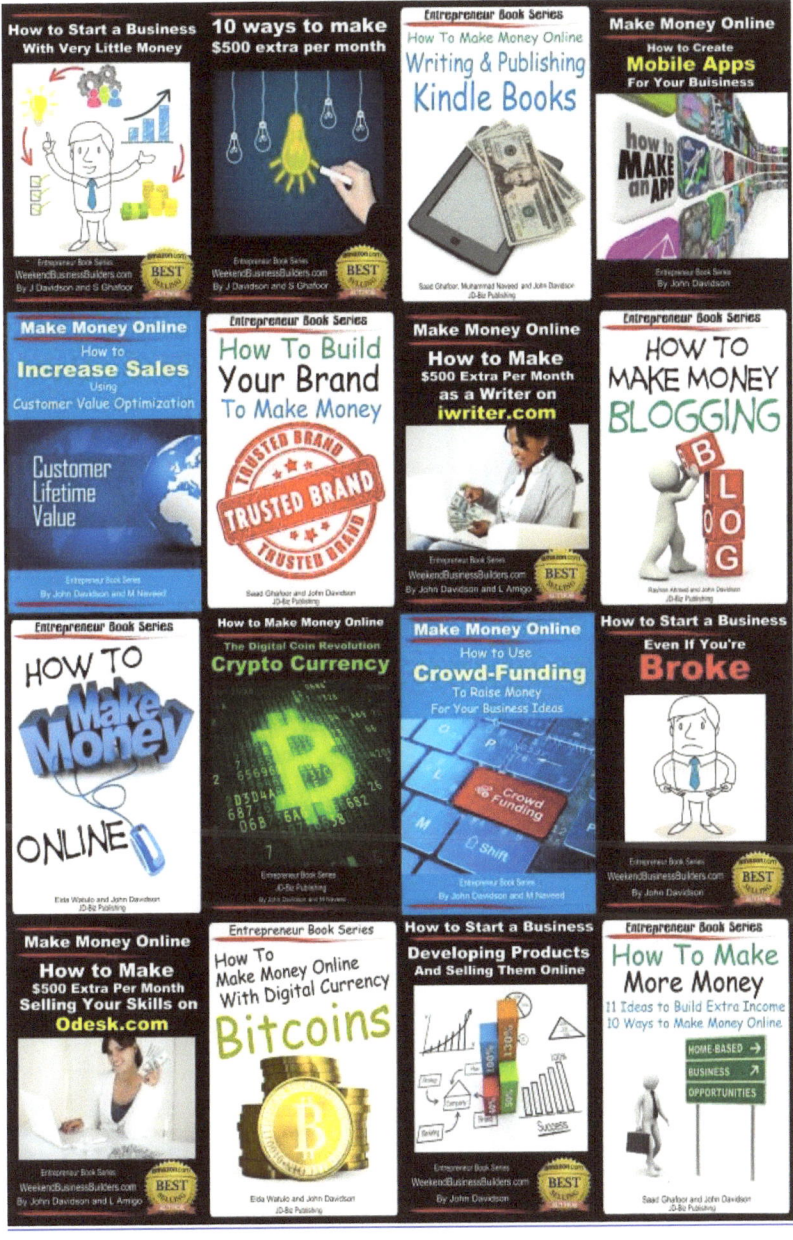

Our books are available at

1. Amazon.com

2. Barnes and Noble

3. Itunes

4. Kobo

5. Smashwords

6. Google Play Books

Download Free Books!

http://MendonCottageBooks.com

Publisher

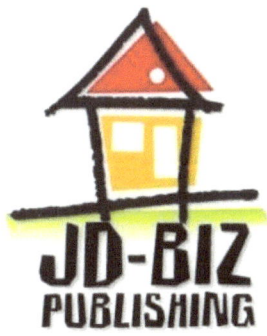

JD-Biz Corp

P O Box 374

Mendon, Utah 84325

http://www.jd-biz.com/

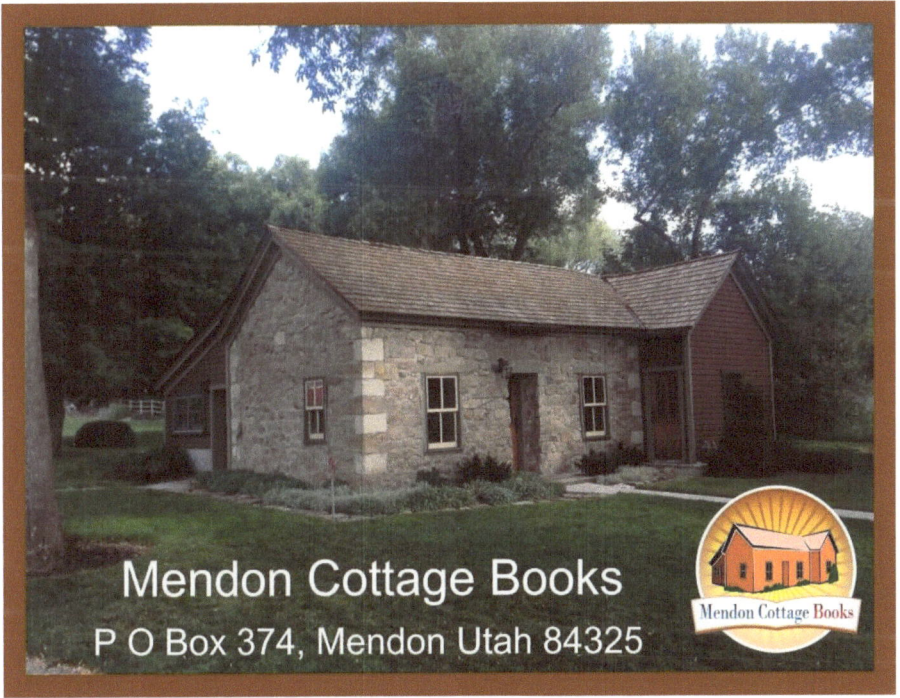